The Ultimate Keto Diet Lunch Cookbook

50 Low-Carb and High Fat Recipes to Lose Weight Fast, Suitable for Women Over 50

Katie Attanasio

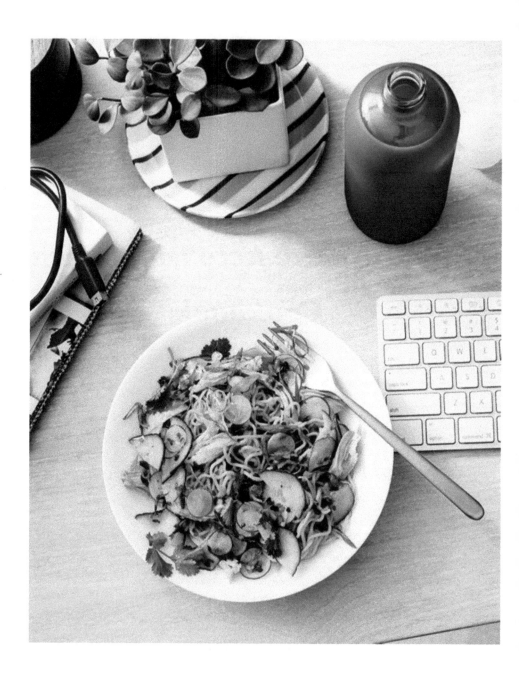

a result of the use of information contained within this document, including, but not limited to, — errors, omissions, or inaccuracies.

Table of Contents

50 Tasty Keto Recipes

1   Chili Lime Steak Fajitas with Squash & Peppers

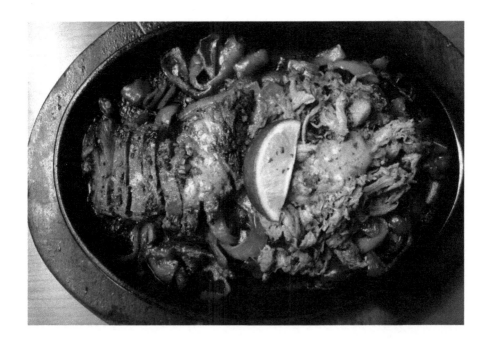

Servings: 4 | **Time:** 30 mins | **Difficulty:** Easy

Nutrients per serving: Calories: 482 kcal | Fat: 32g | Carbohydrates: 11g | Protein: 39g | Fiber: 3g

Ingredients

For the Fajitas:

½ tsp. chili powder

½ tsp. cumin

½ tsp. paprika

1 ½ pound skirt steak membrane removed

1 ½ Tbsp. fresh lime juice

1 ½ tsp. pink Himalayan salt

2 Tbsp. olive oil

2-3 garlic cloves finely minced or For the Veggies:

2 zucchinis sliced in ½" rounds

1 yellow squash sliced in ½" rounds

½ purple onion sliced

1 poblano pepper seeded and sliced into strips

1 colored bell pepper seeded and sliced into strips

3 Tbsp. olive oil

½ tsp granulated garlic

1 ½ tsp. pink Himalayan salt

½ tsp. pepper

¼ tsp. cumin

Method

1.   Combine the chili powder, cinnamon, cumin, paprika, and granulated garlic in a small cup, if necessary. To mix, stir well. In both ends, brush the seasoning generously over the skirt steak, rubbing it in. Place the steak in a ziptop bag and, if used, apply the fresh garlic, olive oil, and the juice. Cover the bag and shake it to guarantee it is covered with the whole steak. For 30 minutes to 3 hours, refrigerate.

2.   Grill meat until meat is to the perfect doneness, around 3 minutes per hand, over a hot, intense heat. To broil, put the rack near the broiler in the oven and broil until it is charred, between 2-4 minutes on either side. Tent the foil with the grilled beef and let the steak sit for 5-10 minutes. Slice the grain in half and eat with the vegetables.

3.   Preheat the oven to 425°F and set aside and line a large sheet pan with parchment. Combine all vegetables and the next 5 ingredients in a large bowl and toss to cover the veggies. Spread them on the lined sheet pan and bake for 15-20 minutes at 425°F or until needed.

2   Keto Jambalaya with Shrimp & Andouille Sausage

Servings: 6 | **Time:** 30 mins | **Difficulty:** Easy

Nutrients per serving: Calories: 431 kcal | Fat: 28g | Carbohydrates: 11g | Protein: 32g | Fiber: 3g

Ingredients

1 Tbsp. bacon fat

1 cup diced celery

1 cup diced onion

1 cup diced green bell pepper

4 cloves garlic finely chopped

½ tsp. salt

½ tsp. dried thyme

2 tsp. Fiesta Brand Cajun-All Seasoning

½ tsp. paprika

1 pound medium shrimp 41/50, peeled and deveined

3 Tbsp. heavy cream optional

Chopped Green Onions

Chopped Parsley

1 15 oz can diced tomatoes

1 pound andouille sausage cut into ¼-1/2 inch slices then cut in half

1 12 oz package of frozen cauliflower rice

Method

1.　　In compliance with the box directions, cook the cauliflower rice. Push between paper towels to dry while cooling and remove excess vapor. You want the cauliflower rice to be dry, so there is no water in your final bowl. Place aside the cauliflower rice.

2.　　Over medium prepare, heat a large skillet and add the sausage. Cook the sausage until golden brown; take it out of the grill. In the pan, add celery, onion, bell pepper, and ½ tsp of salt and cook for 5-7 minutes or until the onion is translucent and the vegetables are tender. Add garlic and cook, stirring continuously, for another 1-2 minutes.

3.　　Lower the heat to medium and put the sausage back in the pan. To mix, add onions, thyme, Cajun-All, paprika and dry cauliflower rice and stir. Apply the vegetables and sausage to the shrimp and cook until the shrimp is finished, stirring regularly, for about 5 minutes. Apply the milk and mix softly to blend. Top up and eat with sliced green onions and chopped parsley!

3   Blackened Venison Tenderloin with Spicy Brussels Sprouts & Cajun Cream Sauce

Servings: 8 | **Time**: 45 mins | **Difficulty**: Easy

Nutrients per serving: Calories: 319 kcal | Fat: 24g | Carbohydrates: 10g | Protein: 17g | Fiber: 3g

Ingredients

For the Crispy Brussels Sprouts:

¾ tsp. salt

1 tsp. Fiesta Brand Cajun Redfish & Meat Seasoning

1 tsp. Fiesta Brand Cajun-All Seasoning

1 tsp. garlic powder

3 cups Brussels Sprouts washed, trimmed and halved

3 Tbsp. bacon drippings or olive oil

For the Venison:

1 tsp. pink Himalayan salt

2 Tbsp. Fiesta Brand Cajun Redfish & Meat Seasoning

2 Tbsp. salted butter

2 venison tenderloins cleaned & trimmed

3 tsp. garlic powder

For the Cajun Cream Sauce:

¼ cup sliced green onion

½ tsp. Blackened Redfish Seasoning

1 cup heavy cream

1 medium tomato seeded & diced

1/3 cup chicken broth or stock

2 cloves garlic finely minced

2 Tbsp. butter

Method

To Prepare the Brussels Sprouts:

1.   1. Preheat the oven to 400°F. Place halved Brussel sprouts on a sheet pan lined with parchment. Drizzle with olive oil or bacon drippings and scatter with seasonings. Toss sprouts with seasoning and oil to coat. 35-45 minutes or until crispy and browned, put in a 400°F oven.

For the Venison

1.   Prepare the venison when the sprouts are frying. Sprinkle the blackening sauce, garlic and salt generously with the tenderloins and transform them to ensure that they are uniformly covered. Preheat the skillet.

2.   Apply the butter until the pan is healthy and hot and the tenderloins go in as soon as it melts. Cook on each side for around 3-4 minutes and put the skillet in the oven with the tenderloins and cook to the appropriate thickness. The amount of time depends on the size and how you want your tenderloin to be prepared. I like my medium and it took about 7-8 minutes in the oven.

3.   Take the tenderloins out of the pan and let them rest while preparing the cream sauce, loosely coated with foil. Move the skillet cautiously back to medium heat.

To Prepare the Cajun Cream Sauce

1.   Add onion, garlic, tomato, and butter to the pan. Sauté for 2 minutes.

2.   cook until broth is reduced by half.

3.   Simmer by stirring continuously for 4 minutes after adding cream.

To Plate:

1.   Take venison and slice it in sizes between ¼ and ½ inch.

2.   Top with cream, sprouts roasted.

3.   Serve!

4   Mexican Tomato Soup

Servings: 4 | **Time:** 25 mins | **Difficulty:** Easy

Nutrients per serving: Calories: 69 kcal | Fat: 4g | Carbohydrates: 7g | Protein: 1g | Fiber: 2g

Ingredients

¼ medium red onion

¼ red, yellow or orange bell pepper

¼ tsp. chili powder

¼ tsp. cumin

¼ tsp. paprika

½ tsp. granulated garlic

1 ½ tsp. salt

1 cup chicken broth (for vegan or vegetarian use Vegetable broth or stock)

1 fresh jalapeno, halved, deveined and seeded

1 stalk celery peeled or strings removed

1 Tbsp. olive oil (additional for drizzling veggies)

2 tsp fresh lime juice

4 medium vine-ripened tomatoes

Topping Ideas:

Chopped Cilantro

Diced Avocado

Queso Fresco

Shredded Cabbage

Shredded Chicken

Sliced Green

Onion Sour Cream

Thinly sliced radishes

Method

1.   Preheat the oven to 400 ° F and put a sheet of parchment in the pan. Place the tomatoes, celery, onion, bell pepper, and jalapeno on a baking sheet, drizzle with the olive oil and roast for 20-25 minutes in the oven until the skin starts to char and break.

2.   In a blender, put all of the vegetables. Just a note... add just 1/4 to 1/2 of the jalapeno to start if you're worried about the soup being too spicy. To raise the sun, you can always add more! Connect the garlic pellets and the next 7 ingredients. Blend on high for 5-10 seconds for a smooth soup. You may also puree the soup using an immersion blender. In a large bowl or saucepan, place all the ingredients and blend until the perfect consistency is reached, creating a soup with a little more texture. Top with the toppings needed and enjoy!

5   Keto Mexican Shredded Chicken

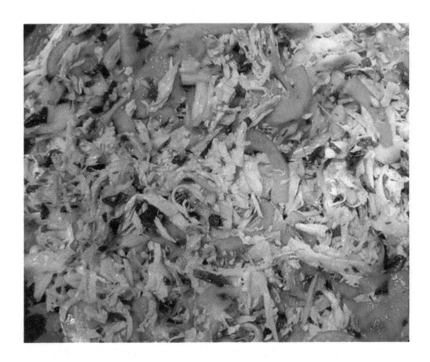

Servings: 8 | **Time**: 20 mins | **Difficulty**: Easy

Nutrients per serving: Calories: 126 kcal | Fat: 9g | Carbohydrates: 5g | Protein: 6g | Fiber: 2g

Ingredients

3 Tbsp. butter

1 Tbsp. chili powder

2 tsp. cumin

2 tsp. granulated garlic

1 Tbsp. paprika

1 tsp. salt

4 cups cooked chicken (dark & white) shredded or pulled

8 oz. tomato sauce

1/2 cup diced onion

1/3 cup chicken stock or water

Method

1.   Melt the butter in a broad skillet over a moderate heat heat and add the chopped onions. Sauté the onions for around 5-7 minutes until they are translucent.

2.   Add the butter, onions, and spices. Cook for the next 30 seconds. Then add the cooked chicken, water and tomato sauce and stir to mix. Switch the heat to low and leave for 5-10 minutes to simmer. When needed, taste and change the seasoning. If you've used water rather than stock, you can need more salt.

3.   Serve hot.

6   Chicken Verde Enchilada Soup

Servings: 6 | **Time:** 1 hr | **Difficulty:** Easy

Nutrients per serving: Calories: 252 kcal | Fat: 17g | Carbohydrates: 7g | Protein: 18g | Fiber: 0g

Ingredients

Verde Sauce:

1 poblano

1/2 tsp. salt

1/2 white onion, cut in half

1/4 cup fresh cilantro

1-2 jalapeno peppers, fresh

2 tbsp. lime juice (about two lime)

4 large garlic cloves

5 tomatillos

For the Soup:

1 cup chopped celery

1 cup chopped onion

1 tbsp. butter

1 tsp. cumin

1/2 cup heavy cream

1/3 cup sour cream

2 quarts chicken broth

2 tsp salt

2 tsp. minced garlic

2/3 cup diced yellow bell pepper

3 cups shredded chicken**

Topping:

Avocado Slices

Chopped Cilantro

Monterrey Jack Cheese

Method

To make the Verde Sauce:

1. Preheat the furnace to 350 °F. Place the poblano, tomatillos, onion, and jalapeno on a sheet pan lined with parchment. In a small piece of foil, wrap your garlic cloves and drizzle the cloves with oil.

2.   Wrap them up and position them with the veggies on the sheet pan. Drizzle with olive oil on the remaining vegetables and roast in the oven for 35-30 minutes or until the peppers are blistered and slightly charred. Set to cool aside.

3.   Seed the peppers and put them in a blender with the onion, tomatillos, garlic cilantro, cloves, lime juice and salt when the vegetables are cool.

4.   Taste the peppers first to test the heat or start with 1/2 a jalapeno at a time and increase to the desired heat level to ensure that your sauce is not too spicy. Mix well until the sauce is smooth. Set aside.

To prepare the soup:

1.   Melt the butter over medium heat in a big stockpot. Add the celery, onion, pepper, and salt to the pot and sauté for 5-7 minutes over medium heat or until the veggies begin to soften. Put the garlic and cumin and cook for a further 2 minutes.

2.   Add the vegetables to the chicken stock and simmer for 20 minutes. To the stock and vegetable mixture, add 1 cup of the prepared Verde sauce, cream and the chicken and whisk to combine. Simmer for 10 more minutes. Remove and stir in the sour cream from the sun. Taste the salt and change it if necessary. Serve immediately with slices of avocado, Monterrey Jack Cheese, sliced cilantro and wedges of lime.

3.   It makes perfect leftovers with this soup! Reheat it gently.

7   Bayou Shrimp Salad with Avocado

Servings: 4 | **Time:** 15 mins | **Difficulty:** Easy

Nutrients per serving: Calories: 493 kcal | Fat: 38g | Carbohydrates: 13g | Protein: 26g | Fiber: 8g

Ingredients

2 cups shrimp

1 lemon

1/2 cup celery, finely diced

2 avocados halved

2 scallions, thinly sliced

3 Tbsp. Fiesta Cajun All Seasoning

8 cups water

1 tbsp. fresh lemon juice

1 tsp. hot sauce, Louisiana or Tabasco

1/2 cup mayonnaise your favorite

1/2 tsp. Fiesta Cajun All Seasoning

1/2 tsp. Worcestershire sauce, gluten-free

1/8 tsp. granulated garlic

2 1/2 tsp. brown mustard

Method

1.   Combine the mayonnaise in a small bowl and the next 6 ingredients for the sauce and whisk to combine. Cover and put the mixture in the refrigerator until you are ready for use.

2.   Combine 8 cups of water and 3 Tbsp of seasoning with the saucepan. In the water, juice the whole lemon and add the lemons as well. Bring this mixture to a boil and let it boil for 5 minutes over medium heat. Add the shrimp and boil for 2-3 minutes or until pink and done with the shrimp... don't overcook. Drain and move the shrimp into a bowl of ice to cool them down and avoid the cooking process. Peel the shrimp until cold. You can keep the shrimp whole or cut in half... I left the small ones whole and cut the others in half.

3.   Combine the boiled, cooled shrimp, celery, scallion, and sauce in a medium dish. Add diced avocado here, if you are not serving on avocado vessels. Gently throw to mix and serve on lettuce leaves or simply eat up straight! Do not add avocado until ready to eat, if prepared in advance.

8 Loaded Chorizo Burgers with Cilantro Lime Crema

Servings: 6 | **Time**: 35 mins | **Difficulty:** Easy

Nutrients per serving: Calories: 473 kcal | Fat: 40g | Carbohydrates: 0g | Protein: 26g

Ingredients

Chorizo Burger Mix

1 pound ground beef (80/20 or 73/27)

1 pound ground pork

1 Tbsp. kosher salt

2 tsp. apple cider vinegar

2 tsp. garlic powder (granulated)

3 Tbsp. water

6 Tbsp. Bolner's Fiesta Brand

Chorizo Mix

Cilantro Lime Crema

1 Tbsp. fresh lime juice,

1 Tbsp. chopped cilantro

salt & pepper to taste

1/2 tsp. garlic powder (granulated)

1/4 cup sour cream, full fat

1/4 cup mayonnaise (your favorite)

Optional Burger Toppings

iceberg or butter lettuce

low carb / keto / gluten-free burger buns

Monterrey Jack Cheese

pickled jalapenos

sliced avocado or guacamole sliced

red onion

sliced tomato

Method

1.   In a big bowl, combine all the burger ingredients together and mix well to mix all the seasonings with the ground meat. Place the mixture in a large zip-top bag and cool for at least 4 hours, but it is best for 12-24 hours!

2.   Remove the mixture of the burger from the fridge and break into 6 portions and shape a patty for each piece. Season with salt and pepper on both sides and leave to sit for 10 minutes.

3.   Over medium heat, preheat a large skillet. Cook 3 patties for around 4-5 minutes per side at a time. Top with cheese if desired and cover for 1 minute with a lid to allow the cheese to melt.

4.   Combine all 6 of the crema ingredients and blend to combine. Season with salt and pepper to taste.

5.   On a bed of lettuce or on your favorite toasted bun, serve up these beautiful burgers. Top with sliced avocado or guacamole, sliced onion, new tomato, and cream and enjoy!

9   Tangy Cucumber Salad With Feta & Dill

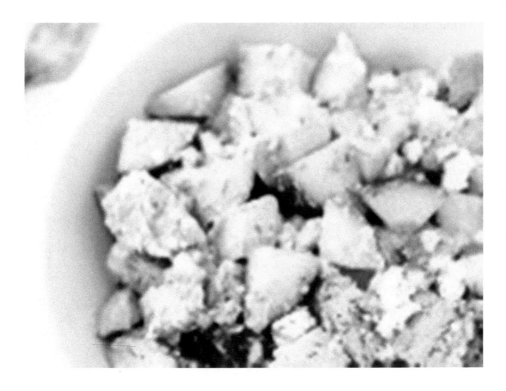

Servings: 3-4 | **Time:** 15 mins | **Difficulty:** Easy

Nutrients per serving: Calories: 660 kcal | Fat: 60g | Carbohydrates: 7g | Protein: 13g | Fiber: 7g

Ingredients

1 large English cucumber, sliced or diced

1 ripe avocados, peeled & diced

1 Tbsp Rodelle's Sesame

Dill Seafood Seasoning

Fresh Dill (optional)

1/2 cup grape or cherry tomatoes, halved

1 1/2 T fresh lemon juice or white wine vinegar

1/2 tsp salt

1/3 cup Feta cheese

1/4 medium purple onion, thinly sliced

1/4 cup olive oil

1/4 tsp Dijon mustard

1/4 tsp black pepper

1/4 tsp garlic powder

Method

1.   In a wide bowl, mix the first 5 ingredients and toss to blend. Whisk together the oil, lime juice / vinegar, the mustard, and the next four seasonings in a small bowl. Pour the dressing over the vegetables, toss and coat gently. Before serving, refrigerate for at least 2 hours. Garnish with fresh chopped dill for extra dill flavor before serving.

2.   Prepare without the avocado if you are cooking and serving the next day, and substitute the avocado around 2 hours before serving.

10   Roasted Vegetable Salad

Servings: 6 | **Time:** 1 hr | **Difficulty:** Easy

Nutrients per serving: Calories: 210 kcal | Fat: 17.3g | Carbohydrates: 9g |Fiber: 5g

Ingredients

½ medium onion, cut into 1" wedges

½ tsp. granulated garlic

1 bell pepper, cut in ½" dice

1 head cauliflower, cleaned and cut into florets

1 small eggplant or about 1 1/2 cups, peeled and diced in 1" cubes

1/2 cup olive oil

10 asparagus spears, cut into 2" pieces

2 small turnips, wedged or diced

2 squash (zucchini or summer), sliced in ½" slices

20 radishes, cut in half if large

3 cups fresh broccoli florets

4T. of basil pesto, heaping (homemade or your favorite brand)

Salt & Pepper

Shredded or shaved Parmesan cheese

Method

1.   Line the two large parchment sheet pans. On one saucepan and radishes, turnips and cauliflower on the other, put squash, bell pepper, broccoli, onion, eggplant, and asparagus.

2.   Drizzle 1⁄4 cup of olive oil into each pan of vegetables. Sprinkle with 1⁄4 tsp of garlic in each pan and usually season vegetables with salt and pepper and toss to cover.

3.   In the oven, put the pans and roast for 30-45 minutes at 425°F or until the veggies begin to brown and caramelize. The broccoli and squash pan will finish first and it will take a little more time to pan with the cauliflower. Do not hurry this segment... this makes the veggies so incredibly delicious! Place them all in a wide bowl, add the basil pesto and toss to coat until all the veggies are done.

4.   Sprinkle with Parmesan cheese and serve at room temperature or high!

11   Chicken Poblano Chowder

Servings: 4 | **Time:** 45 mins | **Difficulty:** Easy

Nutrients per serving: Calories: 660 kcal | Fat: 60g | Carbohydrates: 7g | Protein: 13g | Fiber: 7g

Ingredients

¼ Tsp. chili powder

¼ Tsp. pepper

½ Tsp. cumin

¾ Tsp. salt

1 ½ Tbsp. cornstarch (optional)

1 large carrot, diced

1 medium onion, chopped

1 quart chicken stock

1/8 Tsp. poultry seasoning

2 cups shredded or diced chicken

2 poblano peppers, seeded, deveined & diced

2 Tbsps. butter

3 cloves garlic, chopped

3 oz. cream cheese, softened

3 stalks celery, chopped (about 1 cup)

3 Tbsps. heavy cream

Method

1.   Melt the butter over medium heat in a saucepan.

2.   Add the celery, garlic, carrot, onion, and peppers and sauté for 7-10 minutes or until the onion is translucent. For 2-3 more minutes, add salt, pepper, cumin, poultry seasoning, and chili powder and continue cooking.

3.   Stir in the cream cheese and continue stirring until it is fully melted. To mix, add the chicken stock and stir well. Bring the mixture to a boil, add the chicken and continue to cook for 15-20 minutes until the vegetables are tender.

4.   Whisk the cornstarch and cream together if you are using cornstarch for a slightly thickened soup. When the soup is up to a boil and the vegetables are soft, whisk the cornstarch/cream slurry continuously into the simmering soup. Carry the soup back to a boil to thicken completely. To taste and serve, add salt and pepper!

5.   If you do not use cornstarch, apply the cream to the soup when the vegetables are tender and stir to mix. Salt to taste and eat with mustard! Add avocado, sour cream or chopped cilantro to garnish.

12 Tomato and Basil Salad

Servings: 4 | **Time:** 20 mins | **Difficulty**: Easy

Nutrients per serving: Calories: 127 kcal | Fat: 11g | Carbohydrates: 7g | Protein: 1g | Fiber: 2g

Ingredients

¼ Tsp. freshly ground pepper

½ Tsp. fleur de sel

1 small shallot thinly sliced

2 Tbsps. aged balsamic vinegar

2 Tbsps. fresh basil leaves finely sliced

3 Tbsps. extra virgin olive oil

4 medium heirloom tomatoes cut into wedges

Method

1.   Place the sliced shallots in a shallow bowl and cover to mellow their bite for at least 15 minutes with your favorite aged balsamic.

2.   Place the marinated shallots and vinegar on the sliced tomatoes, a splash of olive oil, a sprinkle of fleur de sel, a few slices of freshly ground black pepper and a chiffonade of basil.

13 Watercress & Chicken Soup

Servings: 4 | **Time:** 40 mins | **Difficulty:** Easy

Nutrients per serving: Calories: 295 kcal | Fat: 15g | Carbohydrates: 8g | Protein: 33g | Fiber: 2g

Ingredients

½ pound fresh watercress or two containers of Go Green hydroponic/living watercress, washed and drained

½ Tsp. Red Boat fish sauce

½ Tsp. toasted sesame oil

1 large shallot thinly sliced

1 pound boneless skinless chicken thighs, thinly sliced

1 Tsp. avocado oil ghee, or fat of choice

2 large carrots peeled and sliced into ¼" coins

2 Tsps. coconut aminos

4 large shiitake mushrooms thinly sliced

6 cups bone broth or chicken broth kosher

salt to taste

Method

1.   If you're using live stuff, grab your watercress and cut off the root end. In cold water, rinse the leaves well and dry them in a salad spinner.

2.   Slice the chicken's boneless, skinless thighs into strips and drop them in a bowl. Add the aminos, sesame oil, and fish sauce to the coconut and mix to ensure that the marinade is well distributed.

3.   Heat the avocado oil over medium heat in a large saucepan and cut up the remainder of the vegetables.

4.   Toss in the shallots, carrots, and shiitake mushrooms and a pinch of salt when the pan is warmed. Sauté until softened by the shallots and mushrooms

5.   Pour in the broth and carry over high heat to a boil.

6.   Attach the chicken and bring it all to a boil again. Reduce the heat to low and cook for 5-10 more minutes, or until the chicken is cooked through and the carrots are softened. Boneless, skinless chicken breast can cook quicker than the thighs, so if the carrots are not yet as tender as you want them, you may need to fish out the chicken first. Thighs, on the other hand, are more forgiving if you overcook them, so once the carrots are cooked through, you should leave them in the pot.

7.   Remove the heat from the pot and stir the watercress into it. Season to taste with more salt and/or fish sauce as soon as the watercress has wilted.

14   Instant Pot Cowboy Chili

Servings: 8 | **Time:** 1 hr 30 mins | **Difficulty**: Easy

Nutrients per serving: Calories: 520 kcal | Fat: 34g | Carbohydrates: 10g | Protein: 47g | Fiber: 3g

Ingredients

For the chili:

1 cup bone broth or chicken broth

1 medium yellow onion cut into ½-inch dice

1 ounce unsweetened chocolate shaved

1 Tbsp. dried oregano

1 Tbsp. smoked paprika

2 Tbsps. ground cumin

2 Tbsps. tomato paste

2 Tsps. Diamond Crystal kosher salt use

1 Tsp. if Morton's brand

3 Tbsps. ancho chili powder

4 garlic cloves peeled and minced

14.4 cups beef chuck roast cut into 2-inch cubes

4 slices bacon cut into ¼-inch pieces

Freshly ground black pepper

Juice from ½ small lime

For the garnish:

½ cup julienned radish

½ cup minced fresh cilantro

½ medium white onion cut into ¼-inch dice

2 limes cut into wedges

plain full-fat coconut yogurt optional

Method

1.   Toss the beef with the salt in a large bowl and set it aside.

2.   Switch on your Instant Pot's sauté feature and throw in the sliced bacon. To ensure browning, stir the bacon regularly.

3.   Move them to a paper-towel once the bacon bits are crunchy.

4.   Throw in the tomato paste and onion and sauté until the onions are tender, around 2-3 minutes.

5.   Meanwhile, in a small bowl or measuring cup, mix the oregano, ancho chili powder, paprika, cumin, and the broth. Mix until the chocolate shavings are smooth and then stir them in

6.   Stir in the garlic and chili-chocolate mixture when the onions have softened. Cook until fragrant or for 1 minute.

7.   Add the lime juice, salted beef, and fried bacon. Stir well.

8.   Cook for 35 minutes under high pressure.

9.   Release the pressure when the chili is done cooking.

10.   Taste the stew with salt and pepper and season accordingly. With your favorite garnishes, top up the chili.

15   Instant Pot Oxtail Stew

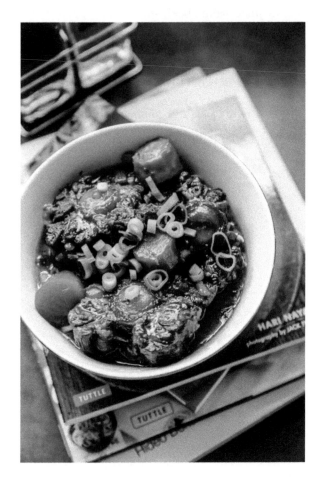

Servings: 8 | **Time:** 1 hr 35 mins | **Difficulty**: Easy

Nutrients per serving: Calories: 767 kcal | Fat: 40g | Carbohydrates: 11g | Protein: 89g | Fiber: 2g

Ingredients

¼ cup minced Italian parsley

1 pound yellow onions finely sliced

1 Tbsp. ghee olive oil, avocado oil, or fat of choice

1 Tbsp. aged balsamic vinegar

1 Tbsp. Red Boat fish sauce

1½ cups marinara sauce I like Rao's brand

3 medium carrots roughly chopped

18 cups oxtails cut crosswise into 3-inch segments

8 garlic cloves peeled and smashed

Freshly ground black pepper

Magic Mushroom Powder or Diamond Crystal kosher salt

Method

1.   In a wide bowl, put the oxtails and add 1 Tbsp. Magic Mushroom Powder.

2.   Toss well and place on a rimmed baking sheet in a single layer.

3.   Under the broiler, pop the oxtails. On each hand, broil for around 5 minutes or until well browned. Alternatively, in the Instant Pot on the "Sauté" feature, you can brown the meat in batches, but it will be tedious and messy.

4. While under the broiler the oxtails are browning, grab your Instant Pot and turn the "Sauté" feature on. Add the ghee or fat of choice when the metal insert is heavy. Toss in the carrots and sliced onions and cook until the onions are softened.

5. Sprinkle with any extra kosher salt or Magic Mushroom Powder. Attach the crushed garlic and stir for approximately 30 seconds or until the garlic is fragrant.

6. Grab the pan with the browned oxtails and nestle them into the vegetables. Pour in some of the pan's stored juices. Mind not to fill more than 2/3rds of your pressure cooker absolutely

7. Pour on the meat with the marinara sauce, fish sauce, and aged balsamic vinegar. Stir well, making sure the bottom of the pot is reached by the liquid.

8. Lock the lid on and program the Instant Pot to cook for 45 minutes under high pressure.

9. Enable the pressure to release naturally when the oxtails are finished cooking. If you are impatient, after 30 minutes have passed, you can release the pressure manually.

10. The meat should fall off the bone and be tender. If required, taste the stew and change the pepper, Magic Mushroom Powder, salt, and/or balsamic vinegar seasoning.

16   Ginger-Scallion Chicken

Servings: 4 | **Time:** 1 hr | **Difficulty**: Easy

Nutrients per serving: Calories: 409 kcal | Fat: 22g | Carbohydrates: 1g | Protein: 48g | Fiber: 1g

Ingredients

¼ cup avocado oil, softened duck fat ghee, or fat of choice

½ cup thinly sliced scallions about 3 scallions

1 Tbsp. grated fresh ginger

1 Tbsp. melted duck fat ghee, or fat of choice

4 chicken breasts bone-in, skin-on (10-12 ounces each)

Diamond Crystal kosher salt

Method

1.   Preheat the oven to 450°F. Add the ginger, scallions, fat, and 2 teaspoons to a small cup of Kosher salt. Mix thoroughly.

2.   Carefully split the skin of each chicken breast away from the meat using your fingers to create a pocket. Now, add 1 Tbsp. the "pesto" under each breast's surface.

3.   Press and rub the skin gently to spread the pesto uniformly. You can continue cooking the chicken at this stage, or refrigerate it for up to a day and roast it later.

4.   Atop a foil-lined baking sheet, place the chicken skin-side up on a wire rack.

5.   Brush the chicken breasts with the melted fat and season with more salt.

6.   Oven-roast for 30 to 35 minutes or until 150°F is inserted into the thickest portion of the chicken registers by an instant-read thermometer.

7.   Give the chicken 5 to 10 minutes to rest. Just serve!

17   Umami Chicken

Servings: 6 | **Time:** 55 mins | **Difficulty**: Easy

Nutrients per serving: Calories: 488 kcal | Fat: 38g | Carbohydrates: 3g | Protein: 32g | Fiber: 1g

Ingredients

⅔ cup plain coconut yogurt or use ½ cup full fat coconut milk

1 Tsp. Red Boat fish sauce

2 Tbsps. lemon juice

2½ Tsps. Magic Mushroom Powder

10.8 cups bone-in skin-on chicken thighs

6 cloves of garlic minced

Method

1.   Mix the Magic Mushroom Powder, coconut yogurt, the garlic, and the fish sauce in a big cup.

2.   Toss in the thighs of the chicken and blend until well coated. Marinate for at least 30 minutes and for up to a day in the fridge.

3.   When you are ready to cook the chicken, heat the oven to 400 ° F convection or 425 ° F traditional. Shake off the excess marinade and place the

chicken on a rimmed baking sheet, skin-side down, on a stainless-steel wire rack.

4.   Roast the chicken for 45 minutes, turn the tray and, at the halfway stage, flip the thighs skin-side up.

5.   When the skin is browned and the chicken's temperature in the thickest part is 165 °F, the thighs are done.

18 Meatza

Servings: 4 | **Time**: 30 mins | **Difficulty:** Easy

Nutrients per serving: Calories: 510 kcal | Fat: 43g | Carbohydrates: 7g | Protein: 23g | Fiber: 2g

Ingredients

¼ cup Castelvetrano olives pitted

¼ cup marinara sauce

¼ pound cremini mushrooms

½ cup goat cheese or almond ricotta

1 pound bulk mild Italian sausage

1 small red bell pepper

1 small red onion

Method

1.   On the parchment, layer the bulk sausage, and use your hands to turn the meat into a rectangle.

2.   Press sausage on parchment paper. Then, using a rolling pin, flatten the sausage evenly until it is around ¼-inch thick.

3.   Put the baking sheet in the hot oven and bake at 425 °F and at the halfway point for about 10 minutes.

4.   Blot the crust well with towels. Remove the meat crust.

5.   Put a layer of marinara sauce on the crust of the steak, and add your favorite toppings.

6.   Put the meat in the oven and cook for another 5-10 minutes or until the toppings are browned.

7.   Remove from the oven and allow it to rest for 5 minutes.

8.   Serve.

19   Dan Dan Noodles

Servings: 6 | **Time:** 45 mins | **Difficulty**: Easy

Nutrients per serving: Calories: 580 kcal | Fat: 50g | Carbohydrates: 12g | Protein: 23g | Fiber: 4g

Ingredients

For the noodles:

2 Tsps. salt

7.2 cups zucchini

For the chili oil:

½ cup light-tasting olive or avocado oil

½- inch piece of cinnamon stick

1 Tbsp. whole black peppercorns

2 Tbsps. crushed red pepper flakes

For the pork:

½ Tsp. ground black pepper

1 jalapeño

1 Tbsp. extra-virgin olive oil

1 Tsp. salt

4.4 cups ground pork

2- inch piece fresh ginger

3 cloves garlic

For the Sauce:

¼ cup coconut aminos

¼ Tsp. ground black pepper

⅓ cup cornichons

½ Tsp. Chinese five-spice powder

2 Tbsps. tahini or almond butter

2 Tbsps. unseasoned rice vinegar

2 Tsps. toasted sesame oil

garnish: a handful cashews 2–3 scallions pinch coconut sugar

Method

1.   Take noodles and toss with salt in a colander.

2.   Make the oil with chili. Combine the peppercorns, oil, red pepper, and cinnamon. Heat the oil as you cook, over medium-low heat.

3.   Only cook the pork. Heat the oil for 2 minutes in a large skillet over medium-high heat. Peel and grind the ginger as the oil heats, mince the jalapeño, and peel and smash the garlic. Apply the aromatics to

the oil and cook for about 1 minute, until fragrant. Season with the pepper and salt, and cook, breaking up the meat with a wooden spoon, until it is browned, 7-10 minutes. Crumble the pork into the pan.

4.   Make the gravy. Place the sesame oil, tahini, black pepper, and Chinese five-spice in a small bowl while the pork is cooking.

5.   Add the vinegar, aminos, and sugar from the coconut; whisk until mixed. Set aside.

6.   In the pan, coat the meat with sauce.

7.   To the skillet, add the cornichons, toss to combine, and move the meat mixture to a big cup. Over medium-high heat, reheat the skillet. Rinse the zucchini noodles in a clean dish towel under running water, drain well, and dry them.

8.   In the heated pan, add the noodles and stir-fry until hot for 2–3 minutes. Return the meat to the pan and mix with two wooden spoons; allow it to heat.

9.   Remove the cinnamon stick from the chili oil using a slotted spoon and discard it. To cool, set the oil aside. Chop the cashews and scallions.

10.   Break the noodles into separate bowls to serve and cover with a drizzle of chili oil, then sprinkle with scallions and cashews.

20   Big-O Bacon Burgers

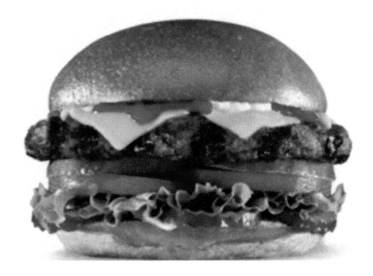

Servings: 4 | **Time:** 30 mins | **Difficulty:** Easy

Nutrients per serving: Calories: 484 kcal | Fat: 41g | Carbohydrates: 3g | Protein: 24g | Fiber: 1g

Ingredients

½ pound cremini mushrooms finely chopped

1 pound ground beef

1½ Tsps. kosher salt

2 Tbsps. ghee lard, or fat of choice, divided

4 ounces bacon frozen and cross-cut into small pieces

Freshly ground black pepper

Method

1.   Take 1 Tbsp Ghee and heat it in a skillet over medium heat.

2.   Sauté the mushrooms. Set the cooked mushrooms aside in order to cool to room temperature.

3.   Combine the bacon, ground beef, and mushrooms in a large bowl and season with salt and pepper. Gently mix the ingredients.

4.   Divide the mixture into four parts and flatten each into 3/4-inch-thick patties using the hands.

5.   Melt the leftover Ghee in a skillet over medium heat, and fry the patties for 3 minutes in the warm fat, turning once.

6.   To allow any excess fat to drain off, move the patties to a wire rack. Pile them with your favorite burger toppings, wrap them in roasted Portobello mushrooms or lettuce leaves, and serve.

21 Cantonese Egg Custard with Minced Pork

Servings: 4 | **Time:** 45 mins | **Difficulty:** Easy

Nutrients per serving: Calories: 228 kcal | Fat: 17g | Carbohydrates: 4g | Protein: 15g | Fiber: 1g

Ingredients

For the filling:

½ pound ground pork or your favorite protein

1 small shallot minced

1 Tsp. ghee

1 Tsp. Red Boat fish sauce

2 Tsps. coconut aminos

3 fresh shiitake mushrooms thinly sliced

3-4 asparagus stalks thinly sliced freshly ground black pepper

For the custard:

¾ cup water

1Tsp. Red Boat fish sauce

3 large eggs

For the garnish:

½ Tsp. toasted sesame oil

2 green onion stalks thinly sliced

2 Tbsps. chopped cilantro

Method

1.   Heat the ghee over a medium-high heat in a large skillet. Break up the pork using a spatula and add shallots to it.

2.   When the shallots are softened, sauté the filling.

3.   Toss in the chopped mushrooms of asparagus and shiitake and stir-fry for about a minute or until the asparagus turns pink.

4.   Season the meat and vegetables with the coconut, fish, and freshly ground pepper sauce.

5.   Next, put cooked meat and vegetables in a shallow bowl.

6.   With approximately two inches of water, fill a large stockpot. In the coated kettle, boil water.

7.   Making the egg custard by mixing the eggs and water as the water in the steamer comes to a boil.

8.   Add 1 Tsp. Sauce with fish and whisk to mix.

9.   Over the meat and vegetables filling, pour the egg mixture.

10.   Place the egg custard carefully in the pot.

11.   For 15-20 minutes or until the custard is fully set, replace the lid on the pot and steam.

12.   Sprinkle with sesame oil and garnish with chopped fresh cilantro and green onions over the savory egg custard.

22   Lamb with Spinach Sauce

Servings: 2 | **Time**: 4 hrs | **Difficulty:** Easy

Nutrients per serving: Calories: 511 kcal | Fat: 37g | Carbohydrates: 14g | Protein: 32g | Fiber: 7g

Ingredients

¼ Cup full-fat coconut milk

½ cup diced tomatoes

1 tbsp. Diamond Crystal kosher salt

1 tbsp. ground cumin

1 tbsp. Lemon juice or more to taste

1 tsp. Ground turmeric

1½ tbsps. Garam masala

2 medium onions thinly sliced

2 tbsps. Ghee

2 tbsps. Ground coriander

3 tbsps. Minced ginger

30 ounces frozen spinach defrosted and squeezed dry

4 garlic cloves minced

14.4 cups lamb necks, cut into 1½ inch cubes, cut crosswise into 2-inch pieces or 7.2 cups of boneless lamb shoulder

---

Freshly ground black pepper

Method

1.   Preheat the oven to 300 °F . Meanwhile, heat the ghee over medium-high heat in a Dutch oven.

2.   With paper towels, dry the lamb necks well and sprinkle with 1 Tsp. Kosher salt.

3.   Sear the lamb in batches in fat until browned on all sides.

4.   Take the browned lamb to a dish and reduce the heat to low. To the empty pan, add the onions and sauté until translucent and smooth (about 10 minutes).

5.   Add the ginger, garlic, coriander, cumin, and turmeric when the onions are soft and whisk until fragrant.

6.   Add the coconut milk and tomatoes and cook until the sauce has thickened. Using the stick blender to mix the sauce until smooth.

7.   Nestle the sauce with the browned lamb parts and add boiling water about 2 cups. Stir in 2 teaspoons. of kosher salt and bring to a boil the contents.

8.   Place the pot in the oven for 2½ hours or until the meat is tender.

9.   Mix the defrosted spinach and garam masala and stir. Cook until the spinach is soft, over medium heat.

10.   Change the salt and pepper and apply the lemon juice to the seasoning.

23   Spicy Ethiopian Chicken Stew

Servings: 6 | **Time:** 2 hrs | **Difficulty:** Easy

Nutrients per serving: Calories: 660 kcal | Fat: 25g | Carbohydrates: 6g | Protein: 32g | Fiber: 1g

Ingredients

¼ cup ghee

¼ Tsp. Freshly ground black pepper

¼ Tsp. ground cardamom

1 Tbsp. berbere seasoning

1 Tbsp. minced ginger

2 cups chicken broth

2 medium red onions thinly sliced

2 Tbsps. freshly squeezed lime juice optional

3 garlic cloves minced

10.8 cups chicken drumsticks skin on or off

4 hardboiled eggs

Diamond Crystal kosher salt

Method

1.   Apply slat to the drumsticks thoroughly and set aside.

2.   Heat the ghee over medium heat in a big Dutch oven. Put the sliced onions and let them cook for 1 to 2 minutes, uninterrupted. To ensure even cooking, season liberally with salt, and gently turn over the pile of onions every 3 to 4 minutes.

3.   Until the onions are softened and greatly reduced in volume, switch the heat to medium-low for approximately 15 minutes.

4.   Cook for another 40 minutes to turn the onions golden brown.

5.   Stir in the caramelized onions with the garlic and ginger, and cook until fragrant, about 30 seconds.

6.   Garnish with cardamom, Berber, and black pepper. Cook the spices until they are fragrant, then add the chicken stock in and stir well to blend.

7.   Nestle the drumsticks into the liquid and carry to a low simmer the contents of the jar. Cover and cook, sometimes rotating the drumsticks, for 45 minutes or until the meat is tender and fried.

8.   Take off the lid of the Dutch oven once the chicken is finished and turn the heat up to medium-high. Cook for 5 to 10 minutes until approximately one-third of the liquid is reduced.

9.   Break the eggs that are hard-boiled into wedges. Switch the chicken drumsticks to a serving plate, garnish with wedges of eggs, and top with the spicy sauce.

24 Pressure Cooker Lamb Shanks

Servings: 4 | **Time:** 1 hr | **Difficulty**: Easy

Nutrients per serving: Calories: 711 kcal | Fat: 44g | Carbohydrates: 12g | Protein: 63g | Fiber: 3g

Ingredients

1 cup bone broth

1 large onion roughly chopped

1 pound ripe Roma tomatoes

1 Tbsp. aged balsamic vinegar

1 Tbsp. tomato paste

1 Tsp. Red Boat fish sauce

1/4 cup minced Italian parsley (optional)

2 celery stalks roughly chopped

2 medium carrots roughly chopped

2 Tbsp. ghee divided

3 garlic cloves smashed and peeled

10.8 cups lamb shanks

Diamond Crystal kosher salt

Method

1.   Melt 1 Tbsp. Ghee in a 6-quart pressure cooker over high heat.

2.   Sear the lamb shanks until all sides have browned (8-10 minutes).

3.   Chop up the onion, celery, carrots, and tomatoes while the lamb is browning.

4.   Take the lamb out of the pot and put it on a plate.

5.   Lower the heat.

6.   Season with salt and pepper and add the celery, carrots, and onion to the pot.

7.   Add the tomato paste and garlic cloves once the vegetables have turned translucent and mix for one minute.

8.   Along with the tomatoes, add the shanks back into the pot and pour the fish sauce, bone broth, and balsamic vinegar in.

9.   Grind on some fresh pepper before locking on to the lid.

10.   Bring the contents of the pot up to high pressure.

11.   Maintain low heat to achieve high pressure for 45 minutes.

12.   When you finish cooking the braised shanks, let the pressure drop naturally.

13.   Plate the shanks and change the seasoning sauce. Ladle shanks with the sauce.

14.   Mince the Italian parsley on top of the braised meat and sprinkle with it.

25 Sous Vide Wild Alaskan Cod

Servings: 2 | **Time**: 40 mins | **Difficulty:** Easy

Nutrients per serving: Calories: 499 kcal | Fat: 17g | Protein: 82g

Ingredients

2 Tbsps. coconut oil or fat of choice

2 wild Alaska cod fillets

Aleppo chile finishing

salt Freshly

ground black pepper

Method

1.   Preheat SousVide Supreme to 130°F.

2.   Drop the frozen cod into the bath for 30 minutes from the fridge.

3.   Pull out. Dry them off and season with Aleppo chile salt-finishing and pepper.

4.   Heat up the oil in a high cast-iron skillet.

5.   Sear for 1 minute on either side of the fish. Serve with some baby spinach and guacamole sautéed!

26 Keto Crab Stuffed Mushrooms With Cream Cheese

Servings: 4 | **Time:** 40 mins | **Difficulty**: Easy

Nutrients per serving: Calories: 267 kcal | Fat: 20.44g | Carbohydrates: 4.67g | Protein: 15.31g | Fiber: 0.7g

Ingredients

1 can lump crabmeat, drained (6 ounce can)

1 pinch salt

1 tbsp green onion, minced

1 tsp fresh parsley, minced

1/2 cup finely grated cheddar cheese (divided use)

1/2 tsp garlic, minced

1/4 tsp red pepper flakes

1/4-1/2 tsp lemon zest

2 tbsp mayonnaise

2 tsp lemon juice

2 tsp prepared horseradish

4 ounces cream cheese, softened

8 large white button or brown mushrooms (1/2 pound)

black pepper to taste

Method

1.   Wash and then dry the mushrooms. Make a large hole in it for filling. Place them on a baking tray.

2.   Preheat the oven to 375°F.

3.   Put cream cheese, mayonnaise, horseradish, lemon juice, green onion, parsley, red pepper flakes, and lemon juice. And stir to melt the cream cheese.

4.   Cheddar cheese folded in half and put it in crab. Add seasoning to the taste.

5.   With the filling, stuff the mushrooms and top with the remaining cheddar cheese.

6.   The mushrooms can be refrigerated overnight at this point, and baked the next day.

7.   Carefully cover it in cling film. Continue with the directions for baking when ready.

8.   Add an extra 5-10 minutes of baking time to prepare the mushrooms.

9.   Put water in baking tray to cover mushrooms. Bake mushrooms for 20-25 minutes.

10.   Refrigerate the remaining mushroom in a tight container. Reheat in the microwave or cover with foil and warm for 30 minutes in a 350 °F oven.

27 Sous Vide Lamb Burgers

Servings: 4 | **Time**: 4 hrs 20 mins | **Difficulty:** Easy

Nutrients per serving: Calories: 323 kcal | Fat: 27g | Carbohydrates: 1g | Protein: 19g | Fiber: 1g

Ingredients

1 pound ground lamb

1 Tsp. Table seasoning

Diamond Crystal kosher salt

Freshly ground black pepper

Method

1.   Preheat your SousVide Supreme to 137 ° F

2.   Apply pepper and salt the ground lamb generously. Then, apply the seasoning Table and mix the meat gently to spread the seasoning.

3.   Divide the meat into four patties and then freeze for two hours.

4.   Vacuum seal them after the patties are solidified, two per container.

5.   Put them for about 2 hours at SousVide Supreme. Then, cut out the patties and use paper towels to rinse them.

6.   Arrange the patties on top of a foil-lined tray on a baking rack. Make circular shapes with the help of a kitchen torch.

28 Sous Vide Black Cod Fillets

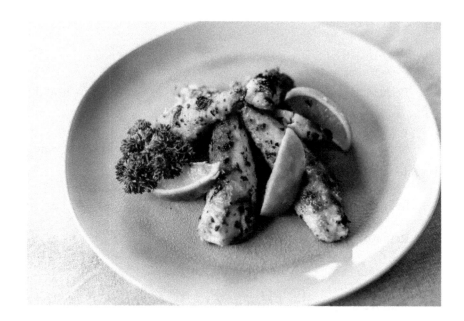

Servings: 3 | **Time**: 1 hr 20 mins | **Difficulty:** Easy

Nutrients per serving: Calories: 352 kcal | Fat: 32g | Carbohydrates: 1g | Protein: 15g | Fiber: 1g

Ingredients

1 cup water

1 pound black cod fillets skin-on and scaled

3 sprigs thyme

3 Tbsp. ghee or fat of choice

4 Tbsp. Diamond Crystal kosher salt

Fleur de sel lemon wedges

Method

1.   Preheat the oven to and use the SousVide Supreme to heat it to 125°F.

2.   Make kosher salt by mixing 2 tbsps. of table salt and 1 cup of water, it will create 10% brine.

3.   Cut each fillet in 2 pieces.

4.   Remove skin and use salt as seasoning on both sides.

5.   Put them in the oven for 35 minutes at 300°F.

6.   Remove the pine bones from the fillets.

7.   In a bag, put the fillets and pour the brine into the mixture. Let them sit in a bowl of ice in the fridge for 10 minutes.

8.   Wash with water and dry the fillets with paper towel.

9.   With a pat of ghee or butter and a thyme sprig, each fillet is vacuum sealed.

10.   Dunk the sealed fillets in the water furnace for 20 minutes.

11.   The skins in the oven should be done. To cool when they are done, remove them from the pan to a wire rack.

12.   When the fillets are finished cooking, place them on a platter and top with the reserved cooking liquid.

13.   On top of the fillets, place fleur de sel, pepper, and a squeeze of fresh lemon juice.

29 Broiled Bacon-Wrapped Tuna Medallions

Servings: 4 | **Time:** 30 mins | **Difficulty:** Easy

Nutrients per serving: Calories: 193 kcal | Fat: 5g | Carbohydrates: 6g | Protein: 32g | Fiber: 1g

Ingredients

¼ cup coconut aminos

¼ cup freshly squeezed orange juice

¼ Tsp. Freshly ground black pepper

½ Tsp. Aleppo pepper (optional)

½ Tsp. Red Boat fish sauce

1 pound tuna albacore loin skinless

1 Tbsp. balsamic vinegar

2 slices bacon thin-cut

Method

1.   Cut the tuna loin crosswise, about 1.5-inch thick, into five mini steaks.

2. Mix coconut amino acids, orange juice, fish sauce, black pepper, Aleppo pepper, and vinegar in a measuring cup. Pour over the fish with the marinade and marinate for 15 minutes.

3. Place the bacon on a plate lined with four sheets of paper towel on a microwave-safe plate and cover with two sheets.

4. For 1-2 minutes, microwave the bacon on high so that it is cooked halfway but still pliable.

5. Wrap a slice of par-cooked bacon with each marinated tuna medallion and put them on a rack on top of a foil-lined baking tray.

6. Broil the bacon-wrapped tuna on one side for about 4 minutes and turn over and cook for an extra 2 minutes.

7. Serve.

30 Lemongrass and Coconut Chicken Drumsticks

Servings: 6 | **Time:** 4 hrs 20 mins | **Difficulty:** Easy

Nutrients per serving: Calories: 319 kcal | Fat: 22g | Carbohydrates: 7g | Protein: 24g | Fiber: 1g

Ingredients

¼ cup fresh scallions chopped

1 large lemongrass stalk

1 large onion thinly sliced

1 thumb-size piece of ginger microplaned

1 Tsp. five spice powder

10 chicken drumsticks skin removed

1¼ cups full-fat coconut milk divided

2 Tbsps. Red Boat fish sauce

3 Tbsps. coconut aminos

4 garlic cloves minced

Diamond Crystal kosher salt

Freshly ground black pepper

Method

1.   Rip off the drumsticks' meat. Put it in a large bowl and season with salt and pepper.

2.   With a grater or beat the stalk and cut finely, trim the fresh lemongrass stalk and grate finely.

3.   Place in a high-powered blender and blitz the garlic, lemongrass, coconut milk, ginger, coconut amino acids, fish sauce, and five spice powder until smooth.

4.   Pour on the chicken with the marinade and blend well.

5.   Dump the onion into the slow cooker's bottom and dump the chicken on top with the marinade. Set low on the slow cooker and cook for 4-5 hours.

6.   Move the chicken and the sauce to a storage container to cool in the fridge for a few days if you're saving it for later. Place the drumsticks in a pot to reheat and bring them to a simmer.

7.   When the stew has finished cooking, remove the chicken and place the sauce and onions in a blender for an extra creamy sauce. Puree the sauce and, at the last moment, pour 1/4 cup more coconut milk into the blender. Return the sauce and chicken to the cooker and keep it warm.

31 Crispy Sous Vide Duck Confit Legs

Servings: 3 | **Time: 1 hr**| **Difficulty**: Easy

Nutrients per serving: Calories: 302 kcal | Fat: 60g | Carbohydrates: 7g | Protein: 13g | Fiber: 7g

Ingredients

2 Tbsps. duck fat

1 package of Grimaud Farms duck

Method

1. For about 45 minutes, put the sealed legs into the SousVide Supreme at 140°F.

2.   Take out the legs and dry them with a pat.

3.   In a cast iron skillet, melt the duck fat over medium-high heat and sear the skin side-down of the legs for around 2 minutes. Flip them over, and brown for about a minute on the other side.

32 Spaghetti and Meatballs

Servings: 4 | **Time:** 25 mins | **Difficulty:** Easy

Nutrients per serving: Calories: 398 kcal | Fat: 34g | Carbohydrates: 5g | Protein: 18g | Fiber: 1g

Ingredients

1 package of kelp noodles or zoodles

1 pound uncooked Italian sausage

1 Tbsp. ghee

12 oz marinara sauce

Method

1.   Make small meatballs of sausage.

2.   Melt one Tbsp. of ghee on medium heat in an iron skillet.

3.   Fry and brown the meatballs in the pan.

4.   Apply about half of Rao's marinara sauce jar and bring to a boil with the sauce.

5.   Cover the pan and cook the sauce for 5 minutes on low heat.

6.   In a colander, put noodles in meatballs and sauce.

7.   Cover and cook for some time, until the noodles are tender.

33 Tuna and Avocado Wraps

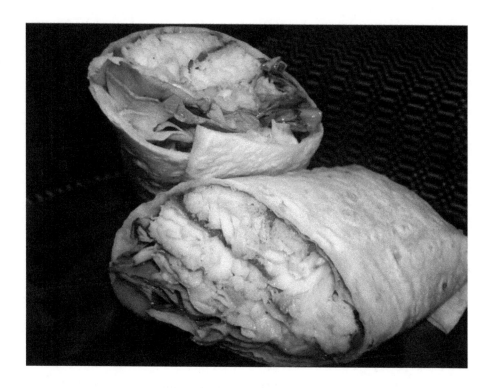

Servings: 1 | **Time:** 15 mins | **Difficulty**: Easy

Nutrients per serving: Calories: 364 kcal | Fat: 19g | Carbohydrates: 14g | Protein: 37g | Fiber: 8g

Ingredients

1 scallion thinly sliced

1/2 jalapeño pepper diced small

1/2 limes

1/2 medium avocado

2 butter lettuce leaves

2 Pure Wraps or toasted nori optional

5 oz canned wild albacore tuna (in water)

Diamond Crystal kosher salt

Method

1. Put tuna in a medium cup and break it gently with a fork.

2. Add Jalapeño and chopped scallions. Then, toss them with the tuna in the tub.

3. Mix in the pepper, the salt, and the lime spritz.

4. Mash half an avocado with salt, pepper, and the remainder of the lime juice in a separate dish.

5. Scoop the guacamole up, add seasoned tuna to the bowl and mix to blend.

6. Grab two Pure Wraps and put on each one a slice of lettuce. Break the lettuce with the tuna salad, roll it up, and serve.

34   Oven-Braised Mexican Beef

Servings: 6 | **Time:** 3 hrs 10 mins | **Difficulty:** Easy

Nutrients per serving: Calories: 379 kcal | Fat: 22g | Carbohydrates: 6g | Protein: 38g | Fiber: 1g

Ingredients

½ cup chicken stock

½ cup minced cilantro optional

½ cup roasted salsa I use Trader Joe's Double Roasted salsa

½ Tsp. Red Boat Fish Sauce

1 medium onion thinly sliced

1 Tbsp. chili powder I use Penzeys Arizona Dreaming

1 Tbsp. coconut oil or fat of choice

1 Tbsp. tomato paste

1½ Tsps. kosher salt Diamond Crystal brand

2 radishes thinly sliced (optional)

2½ pounds boneless beef short ribs beef brisket, or beef stew meat cut into 1½-inch cubes

6 garlic cloves peeled and smashed

Method

1.   Mix the chili powder, cubed beef, and salt in a large cup.

2.   Melt fat in a big dutch oven over medium heat.

3.   Sauté onions until translucent.

4.   Stir in the tomato paste and garlic and cook for 30 seconds.

5.   Add the seasoned beef and add the stock, salsa, and sauce to the fish. Boil it.

6.   Cover the pot and put it in the oven at 300 ° F until the beef is tender, or for 3 hours.

7.   Spoon the beef on a serving dish and cover it with cilantro and/or radishes.

35 Grilled Calamari and roasted Peppers

Servings: 3 | **Time:** 45 mins | **Difficulty:** Easy

Nutrients per serving: Calories: 334 kcal | Fat: 22g | Carbohydrates: 10g | Protein: 24g | Fiber: 1g

Ingredients

1 medium red bell pepper

1 pound squid cleaned and gutted

1 small shallot thinly sliced

1 Tbsp. balsamic vinegar

1/4 cup Italian parsley

2 Tbsp. extra virgin olive oil

2 Tbsp. melted ghee or fat of choice

Diamond Crystal kosher salt

Freshly ground black pepper

Juice from 1/2 a lemon

Method

1.   Place the pepper in a bowl and cover with plastic wrap or foil tightly and steam it for at least 15 minutes.

2.   Rub off the skin that has been blackened and cut the seeds, stem, and ribs.

3.   Break and set aside the bell pepper into thin strips.

4.   Rinse and squid dry. Cut open each one so that it'll lay flat on the grill.

5.   With the cooking fat, put salt and pepper to taste, toss the squid.

6.   In a small cup, mix the thinly sliced shallots with balsamic vinegar and let them mellow out.

7.   Heat up your gas grill. Toss on the squid once it's super-hot and cook on each side for 20-30 seconds.

8.   Cut them up and throw them in a bowl until the squid is flash-grilled.

9.   Over the squid, add juice from half a lemon and pour in the olive oil.

10.   Toss the sliced peppers, shallots, pepper, and salt into the balsamic-marinated ones.

11.   Mix well with everything and sprinkle with the parsley. Taste and change as required for seasoning.

36 Chicken Spaghetti Squash Bake

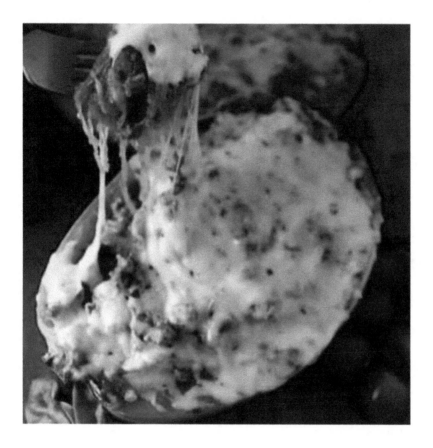

Servings: 6 | **Time:** 1 hr 50 mins | **Difficulty:** Easy

Nutrients per serving: Calories: 553kcal | Fat: 42g | Carbohydrates: 12g | Protein: 30g | Fiber: 2g

Ingredients

1 whole spaghetti squash

2 ounces cream cheese

2 Tbsps. butter

6 ounces cheddar, shredded

3 ounces mozzarella, shredded

3 cups cooked, shredded chicken

2 cloves garlic, minced

1 Tsp. onion powder Chives, for garnish

1/2 Tsp. ground mustard

1/2 Tsp. pepper

1 1/4 cups heavy whipping cream

10.5 ounces Ro*Tel, drained

Method

To cook the spaghetti squash:

1.   Preheat the oven to 400 °F.

2.   Break the squash in half lengthwise and scoop out the seeds. Dispose of the seeds.

3.   Drizzle with olive oil. Cook for 1 hour on a baking sheet in oven or until the squash is tender with a fork.

4.   Follow these instructions to cook in the Instant Pot.

5.   When the squash is cooked, shred the squash by using a fork to scrape the squash widthwise into long spaghetti-like strands.

6.   Place the squash strands in a large mixing bowl.

To make the cheese sauce:

1.   In a medium saucepan, add the cream cheese, heavy cream, and butter and melt them on medium heat.

2.   Whisk the mustard and pepper into the field.

3.   Remove the cheddar and mozzarella from the heat and whisk until the mixture is smooth. To assemble:

1.   Heat the oven to 350 °F. With non-stick spray, spray a baking dish.

2.   To the mixing bowl with the spaghetti squash, add the chicken, garlic, and onion powder.

3.   To coat, pour the cheese sauce over the top and stir gently.

4.   In the prepared baking dish, pour the mixture into it and bake for 20 minutes or until hot and bubbly.

5.   Before serving, sprinkle it with chives.

37 Instant Pot Cajun Ranch Chicken Soup

Servings: 2 | **Time:** 40 mins | **Difficulty:** Easy

Nutrients per serving: Calories: 412 kcal | Fat: 23g| Carbohydrates: 5g | Protein: 44g | Fiber: 1g

Ingredients

½ cup shredded white cheddar

1 1/2 pounds chicken breast

1 jalapeno, minced, see note

1 Tsp. dried chives

1 Tsp. dried dill

1 Tsp. dried parsley

1 Tsp. onion powder

2 cups baby spinach

2 cups reduced sodium chicken broth

2 Tsps. Cajun seasoning, more as needed

3 cloves garlic

4 slices bacon, diced

8 ounces cream cheese

Cilantro, jalapeno slices, green onions, for garnish

Method

1.   Add bacon to the pot and cook till it becomes crisp.

2.   Pour the broth into the pot.

3.   To mix, add the garlic, chicken, Cajun seasoning, jalapeno, parsley, dill, and chives to the pot and stir.

4.   Cover, close the vent, and cook for 18 minutes under high pressure. Enable 10 minutes to relieve the pressure naturally.

5.   Remove the chicken from the pot and use two forks to shred it.

6.   In a small cup, microwave the cream cheese.

7.   Add the cream cheese and set the pot to sauté. Whisk well until the soup has completely melted into the cream cheese.

8.   Put the chicken along with the spinach and cheddar back in the pot.

9.   Ladle it into bowls and serve, if needed, with jalapeno, cilantro, and green onions.

38   Keto Chicken Fajita Soup

Servings: 6 | **Time**: 38 mins | **Difficulty**: Easy

Nutrients per serving: Calories: 392 kcal | Fat: 26g | Carbohydrates: 11g | Protein: 29g | Fiber: 4g

Ingredients

½ Cup chopped cilantro

½ tsp. Chili powder

1 fresh lime, juiced

1 medium onion, chopped

1 pound chicken breasts

1 tbsp. Avocado oil

1 tbsp. Chipotles

1 tbsp. Cumin

1 tsp. Salt

2 bell peppers, chopped

Diced avocado,

2 cloves garlic,

minced Cheddar

2 cups chicken broth

Diced tomatoes,

8 ounces cream cheese

Sour cream,

Method

1.   Add the onion and peppers and cook for about 5 minutes.

2.   To coat the vegetables, add the chipotle, garlic, chili powder, cumin, and salt to the pot and mix.

3.   To the pot, add the lime juice, chicken broth, and chicken.

4.   Cover and turn the vent to seal, and cook for 18 minutes at high pressure.

5.   Remove the chicken and use two forks to shred it.

6.   To sauté, turn the Instant Pot on and add the cream cheese.

7.   Put the cilantro and stir well.

8.   Using sour cream, onions, avocado, or cheese to serve.

39   Keto Burrito Bowl

Servings: 1 | **Time**: 5 mins | **Difficulty:** Easy

Nutrients per serving: Calories: 374 kcal | Fat: 25g | Carbohydrates: 15g | Protein: 27g | Fiber: 6g

Ingredients

1 cup Mexican Cauliflower Rice

1 Tbsp. chopped cilantro

1/2 cup Mexican Shredded Beef

1/4 cup Keto Guacamole

1/4 cup Pico de Gallo

1/4 cup shredded cheddar cheese

Method

1.   Mix ingredients in a small bowl and season to taste.

2.   Add pepper and salt or hot sauce (optional).

3.   Serve.

40 Dill Pickle Egg Salad Sandwiches

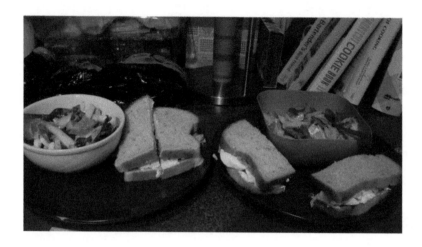

Servings: 3 | **Time:** 30 mins | **Difficulty:** Easy

Nutrients per serving: Calories: 465 kcal | Fat: 35g | Carbohydrates: 7g | Protein: 30g | Fiber: 1g

Ingredients

For the egg salad:

½ cup chopped dill pickles

1 Tbsp. dill pickle juice

1 Tbsp. fresh dill

1 Tbsp. prepared yellow mustard

3 Tbsps. Mayonnaise

6 hard boiled eggs

Salt and pepper, to taste

For the chaffles:

1 1/2 cups finely shredded mozzarella

1 Tbsp. coconut flour

3 eggs, beaten

3/4 Tsp. baking powder

Method

To make the egg salad:

1.   Peel and cut into small bits with the shells.

2.   Including the rest of the ingredients, add the eggs to a bowl and mix.

3.   serve or store in fridge. To make the chaffles:

1.   To preheat, connect the waffle iron to electricity.

2.   Whisk the coconut flour, eggs, and baking powder together. Mix the mozzarella.

3.   To cover the bottom of the waffle iron, spoon just enough batter and close the waffle iron.

4.   For 3 minutes, cook. Remove the waffle and repeat until you have 6 chaffles fried, with the remaining batter.

To assemble:

1.   Divide the egg salad evenly between three chaffles.

41   Bruschetta Chicken

Servings: 4 | **Time:** 45 mins | **Difficulty**: Easy

Nutrients per serving: Calories: 355 kcal | Fat: 18g | Carbohydrates: 6g | Protein: 45g | Fiber: 1g

Ingredients

For the chicken:

½ Tsp. salt

1 Tsp. Italian seasoning

2 cloves garlic, minced

2 Tbsps. balsamic vinegar

2 Tbsps. olive oil

3/4 cup shredded mozzarella

4 chicken breasts, about 6 ounces each

For the bruschetta:

½ cup chopped basil

½ small red onion, chopped

½ Tsp. salt

1 ½ cups cherry tomatoes, halved

1 Tsp. balsamic vinegar

1 Tsp. olive oil

3 cloves garlic, minced

Method

1.   Add the chicken breasts in baking dish.

2.   In a small cup, add the balsamic vinegar, oil, Italian seasoning, garlic, and salt. Whisk them to mix. Place the chicken over it and switch to coat it.

3.   While the oven heats to 425 ° F, let the chicken set for 10 minutes.

4.   Put the chicken in the oven and bake until the chicken reaches 165 ° F or for 25-30 minutes.

5.   Blend all ingredients for the bruschetta to a bowl.

6.   Remove from the oven when the chicken is baked, and top with the mozzarella.

7.   To melt the cheese and warm the tomatoes, pour the bruschetta over the chicken and return to the oven for 5 minutes.

42   Crispy Baked Chicken Thighs

Servings: 2 | **Time**: 50 mins | **Difficulty**: Easy

Nutrients per serving: Calories: 796 kcal | Fat: 54g | Carbohydrates: 2g | Protein: 80g | Fiber: 0g

Ingredients

½ Tsp. cracked pepper

1 Tsp. chopped parsley

1 Tsp. garlic powder

1 Tsp. onion powder

1 Tsp. paprika

1 Tsp. salt

2 Tbsps. avocado oil

3 pounds bone-in chicken thighs

Method

1.   In a big zip top bag, add all the ingredients except for the parsley and seal them. Smush the chicken in bag to season it.

2.   On the baking sheet, arrange the chicken and bake 400°F for 35-45 minutes.

3. sprinkle the chicken with parsley.

4. Serve.

43   Baked Salsa Chicken

Servings: 4 | **Time:** 45 mins | **Difficulty**: Easy

Nutrients per serving: Calories: 216 kcal | Fat: 11g | Carbohydrates: 4g | Protein: 22g | Fiber: 2g

Ingredients

½ Tsp. chili powder

½ Tsp. cumin

1 ½ cups salsa

1 cup shredded pepper jack cheese

1 Tbsp. chopped cilantro

1 Tsp. garlic salt

4 chicken breasts, about 6 ounces each

Method

1.   Pound the breasts of the chicken to an even size.

2.   Add the chili powder, garlic salt, and cumin to the chicken seasoning.

3.   Add ½ cup of salsa and spread to cover the bottom of dish.

4.   On top of the salsa, put the chicken. Then, pour the remaining salsa over it.

5.   Bake for 30 minutes at 375 °F, or until the chicken reaches 165 °F.

6.   Sprinkle the top of the chicken with the cheese and remove it from the oven.

7.   For 3-4 minutes, return to the oven to melt the cheese.

8.   Sprinkle with cilantro.

44 Chicken Alfredo Pizza

Servings: 8 | **Time**: 35 mins | **Difficulty**: Easy

Nutrients per serving: Calories: 660 kcal | Fat: 60g | Carbohydrates: 7g | Protein: 13g | Fiber: 7g

Ingredients

For the crust:

¾ cup almond flour

1 egg

2 cups shredded mozzarella

2 Tbsps. cream cheese

For the Alfredo sauce:

1 clove garlic, minced

1 ounce cream cheese

1/3 cup heavy whipping cream

1/4 cup shredded Parmesan cheese

2 Tbsps. Butter

For assembling:

1 cup chicken, cooked and cubed

1/4 cup spinach, chopped

2 cups Mozzarella cheese

Method

To make the crust:

1.   Preheat the furnace to.

2.   Microwave the cream cheese and mozzarella for 1 minute.

3.   Add egg and almonds.

4.   On a large sheet of parchment paper, place the dough. Top it with a second parchment cover.

5.   Roll the dough out into a circle with a diameter of 12 inches.

6.   Take out the top piece of parchment and pass the bottom sheet to a pizza pan with the dough on it.

7.   Bake for 10 minutes at 425 °F or until finely golden in the crust.

To make the Alfredo sauce:

1.   Add the butter, cream, garlic, and cream cheese to a small saucepan over medium heat to melt cheese and butter.

2.   Add parmesan cheese and stir to make it creamy and smooth.

To assemble:

1.   Place the Alfredo sauce uniformly over the crust of the pizza.

2.   Cover the mozzarella cheese with 3/4 of it.

3.   Attach the spinach and chicken and top with the remainder of the mozzarella.

4.   Return for 10 minutes to the oven.

5.   Let set before slicing and serving for 2 minutes.

45 Pork Chops with Dijon Sauce

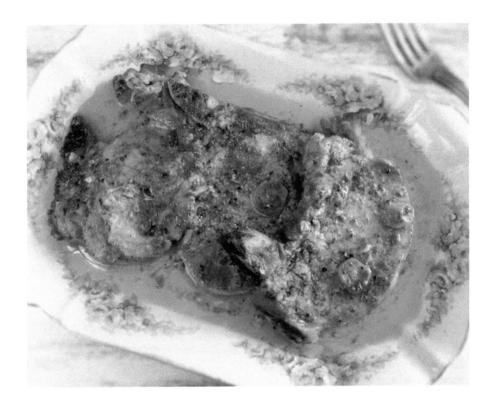

Servings: 4 | **Time:** 17 mins | **Difficulty:** Easy

Nutrients per serving: Calories: 201 kcal | Fat: 17g | Carbohydrates: 1g | Protein: 12g | Fiber: 0g

Ingredients

4 boneless pork chops, about 6 ounces each

1 Tbsp. avocado oil

2 Tbsps. dijon mustard

1 Tsp. minced parsley

1/2 Tsp. salt

1/2 Tsp. cracked pepper

1/3 cup chicken broth

1/3 cup heavy cream

Method

1.　　Sprinkle with salt and pepper on both sides of the pork chops.

2.　　Heat oil over medium heat in a large skillet until it shimmers.

3.　　Add the pork chops to the skillet and cook, about 5 minutes per side, until golden on each side and cooked through.

4.　　Remove the pork chops and set them aside on a tray.

5.　　To scrape up any browned bits from the bottom of the plate, add the chicken broth to the skillet and whisk well.

6.　　Apply the dijon and cream and cook until the sauce reduces and thickens to your liking, stirring frequently.

7.　　Put the pork chops back in the skillet and sprinkle them with parsley.

8.　　Serve over the pork chops with a drizzle of Dijon cream sauce.

46   Baked Chicken Drumsticks

Servings: 6 | **Time:** 50 mins | **Difficulty:** Easy

Nutrients per serving: Calories: 323 kcal | Fat: 18g | Carbohydrates: 1g | Protein: 37g | Fiber: g

Ingredients

2 pounds chicken drumsticks

2 Tbsps. avocado oil

1 Tsp. paprika

1 Tsp. garlic powder

1 Tsp. onion powder

1 Tsp. chopped parsley

½ Tsp. salt

½ Tsp. cracked pepper

Method

1.   In a big zip top bag, add all the ingredients and seal them. Smush the chicken in bag to season it.

2.   On the baking sheet, arrange the chicken and bake 400°F for 45 minutes.

47 Pizza Stuffed Chicken

Servings: 4 | **Time:** 45 mins | **Difficulty**: Easy

Nutrients per serving: Calories: 402 kcal | Fat: 26g | Carbohydrates: 6g | Protein: 32g | Fiber: 1g

Ingredients

¼ cup Parmesan cheese

½ Tsp. Italian seasoning

½ Tsp. salt

1 cup pizza sauce

1 Tsp. garlic powder

1 Tsp. minced parsley

2 cups grated mozzarella, divided

2 Tsps. avocado oil

32 slices pepperoni

4 chicken breasts, about 6 ounces each

Method

1.   Place the chicken breasts on a cutting board.

2.   Drizzle oil on the chicken and season with garlic powder, salt and Italian seasoning.

3.   In the chicken breast, position 1/4 cup of mozzarella. Over the cheese, add 4 slices of pepperoni.

4.   In the prepared baking dish, put the chicken and drizzle it with the pizza sauce. Spread the sauce over the chicken tops to coat them.

5.   Sprinkle the remaining mozzarella with it. Top with the slices of Parmesan and the remaining pepperoni.

6.   Bake chicken for 30-35 minutes at 375°F.

7.   Until serving, sprinkle it with fresh parsley.

48 Low Carb Chicken Patties

Servings: 10 | **Time:** 16 mins | **Difficulty**: Easy

Nutrients per serving: Calories: 373 kcal | Fat: 25g | Carbohydrates: 5g | Protein: 33g | Fiber: 3g

Ingredients

2 cups cooked, shredded chicken breasts

2 Tbsps. mayonnaise

1 egg

2 green onions, minced

1 Tsp. fresh dill

1 Tsp. fresh parsley

1 Tsp. salt

2 Tbsps. butter, for frying

1/2 cup almond flour

1/2 Tsp. pepper

Method

1.   To a mixing bowl, add all the ingredients except for the butter and whisk well to combine.

2.   In order to scoop the mixture into your hand, use a medium cookie scoop.

3.   Heat a large skillet with a heavy bottom over medium heat and add butter.

4.   Add the chicken patties to the skillet once the butter has melted and cook until golden brown on each side, about 3 minutes on each side.

5.   Immediately serve.

49 Ranch Grilled Chicken

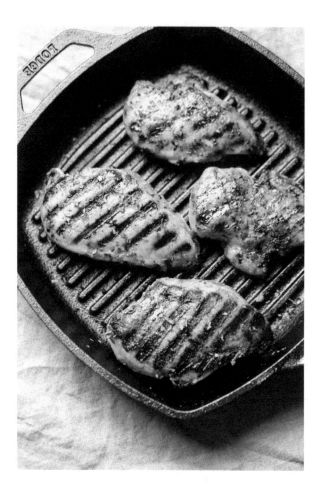

Servings: 6 | **Time:** 8 hrs 20 mins | **Difficulty:** Easy

Nutrients per serving: Calories: 494 kcal | Fat: 19g | Carbohydrates: 4g | Protein: 71g | Fiber: 1g

Ingredients

½ cup avocado oil

½ cup ranch dressing

1 Tbsp. apple cider vinegar

1 Tbsp. chopped parsley

1 Tsp. hot sauce

1 Tsp. salt

2 Tbsps. buttermilk

2 Tbsps. Worcestershire sauce

3 pounds boneless, skinless chicken breasts

Method

1.   To a mixing bowl, add all but the chicken.

2.   Add the chicken breasts and add the marinade to a baking dish or gallon zip top container. To coat the chicken, stir well.

3.   For at least 30 minutes and up to 8 hours, marinate the chicken in the refrigerator. The longer you marinate the chicken, the more delicious it will be.

4.   Heat the grill to a heat that is medium.

5.   Remove the chicken from the marinade and let the chicken drip off a lot of it, then return it to the hot grill.

6.   Grill on each side for 5-10 minutes until cooked through, depending on your chicken's thickness.

50 Lemon Caper Chicken

Servings: 4 | **Time**: 25 mins | **Difficulty**: Easy

Nutrients per serving: Calories: 326 kcal | Fat: 19g | Carbohydrates: 2g | Protein: 36g | Fiber: 0g

Ingredients

¼ cup heavy cream

1 cup chicken broth

1 pound thin sliced chicken breasts

1 Tbsp. avocado oil

1 Tbsp. lemon juice

1 Tsp. pepper

1 Tsp. salt

2 Tbsps. butter

3 Tbsps. capers

Method

1.   With salt and pepper, season the chicken on both sides.

2.   Heat the avocado oil over medium heat in a big, heavy-bottomed skillet.

3.	Cook the chicken, flipping for about 8 minutes halfway through cooking.

4.	Remove the chicken and set it aside on a tray.

5.	Apply the butter and the chicken broth to the skillet and bring it to a boil.

6.	Reduce the chicken broth by half, about 5 minutes or so.

7.	Apply the lemon juice and cream to the skillet and boil until the sauce is thick enough to cover the back of the spoon, stirring occasionally, for around 5 minutes.

8.	Add the sauce to the capers and stir to combine.

9.	Put the chicken back in the skillet and coat it with sauce. To re-warm the chicken, cook for 1 more minute.

10.	Immediately serve.

Lightning Source UK Ltd.
Milton Keynes UK
UKHW020420070521
383233UK00001BA/57